Brain Matters-A True Story of Survival

Brain Matters-A True Story of Survival

Amy J Van Patten Ofenbeck
with Dayna Harpster

ISBN: 1522963146
ISBN 13: 9781522963141

Special Thanks to

My family:
Todd Ofenbeck
Mark and Nancy Van Patten
Raymond "Daddy O" Ofenbeck
Lori Sandquist
Rae Kyriazis

The doctors and nurses who have taken care of me:
Dr. George Sypert
Dr. Joy Arpin
Dr, Gary Correnti
Dr Jaime Alvarez
Dr. William Friedman
Dr. Fred Schaerf
Melissa Schaerf
Kerry Ellis Berry

My physical therapist Abe Abarbanel and all the great therapists at The Center for Rehabilitation and Wellness Ft Myers

My great friends:
Shannon Powell Gargiulo
Ron Palmer
Doug Larson
Jim Rasor

My former co-workers from Waterman Broadcasting:
Bob Goldberger
Kellie Burns
Craig Wolf
Emily Norman
The late Harry Horn
Colleen Gallagher Goldenfarb

All the viewers of WSIL TV3 in Carterville, Illinois

Thanks to my co-writer
Dayna Harpster

Thank you to all those who donated to my GoFundMe account to get this book published

And thank you to Goodwill Industries of Southwest Florida

Gulfshore Life magazine July 2013 "The Underdogs Win" by Cayla Stanley

Amy Ofenbeck
"She was 26, only nine months into her marriage and fresh on the job as an ABC-7 reporter and news anchor for Waterman Broadcasting. The aneurysm was just the first of seemingly endless derailing setbacks. But despite repeated complications and constant challenges, Ofenbeck maintains an infectious optimism."

This book is dedicated to my husband Todd-thank you and I love you with all my heart.

Foreword

by Craig Wolf, Waterman Broadcasting employee from 1993-2011

When Amy Ofenbeck told me she was going to write a book about nearly dying from a brain aneurysm, I knew there'd be plenty of skeptics. I was one of them., After all, there is no more skeptical environment than a TV newsroom, where Amy lived and breathed for most of her professional life and where I first met her almost twenty years ago.

Those skeptics had good reason to be doubtful of her ability to undertake the gargantuan task of writing a book. The intense work, sweaty frustration, and harsh discipline (I myself, am writing numerous books that I haven't written yet) are monumental enough for those who haven't had 8 brain surgeries, been in a coma, fought for our lives and dealt with everything from learning to walk again to even scorn from some of those with whom we once worked.

I was fortunate enough to work closely with Amy's devoted husband Todd. We did a lot of traveling together on stories. Much of what I learned about Amy's horrible and intense struggles came from him on those trips. I've come to the conclusion there must be something in the water at the Ofenbeck household. Because rarely will you come across people that have turned life's proverbial lemon into lemonade as Amy and Todd have. And still strive to do.

Amy went to a place where no one wants to be, but occupies it with grace, a smile and a fierce determination all of us want to possess. While so many of her family and friends were hopeful for Amy's comeback, that became a moot point. Because after Reading her incredible story, you'll realize she never really left.

CHAPTER 1

The Big Day

October 19,1997-It's my first wedding anniversary. What a day to celebrate! And for a time, I'd even forgotten I was married. Something happened at the gym that Tuesday afternoon in July that altered everything.

It was July 15. I had just put in a good day working as a morning anchor and reporter at WZVN TV in Ft Myers, Florida. My husband and I had just started there in December. He was behind the camera I was in front. We were very lucky to get jobs at the same time at the same station. And we were loving it! We loved going to the beach with friends every weekend, we loved being close to my father-in-law, Raymond "Daddy O" we just loved everything about being in Southwest Florida.

I worked that day anchoring the morning news and then reported on and wrote a story. Every day I had to do a story for the evening news but because I worked early mornings it needed to be timeless and undated. This particular day I did a story about wildlife rehabilitation. It was a good story and both my photographer and I were happy with it. I really liked my job and was told I was pretty good at it.

But that particular day after work would be a life changer. I was working out at the gym as usual because I'm a gym rat. I love to exercise. A woman I worked with and I belonged to a women's gym in Ft Myers so we tried to work out together as much as we could. But that day I was there that day lifting weights when all of a sudden I put my hands to my head, sat down on a weight machine and collapsed. I was slipping into unconsciousness, gurgling, my eyes rolling back into my head. These details have been told to me-I remember nothing. I've been told I stopped breathing. Luckily, some nurses and other medical professionals were working out there too and started administering first aid. An ambulance was called and off I went to the nearest hospital. I've been told they suspected a brain injury given my symptoms so I was sent to a hospital that specialized in that.

Someone from the gym ended up calling my friend and co-worker because they had no emergency contact information for me. She rushed to the hospital and I think she ended up calling the station. The message finally got through to my husband. He was out in the field and was just told to come back to the station. They didn't tell him why until he got back. When he got back they told him that I collapsed at the gym and was at the hospital. He says he thought I was just dehydrated and it was no big deal. He remembers that's what he was telling himself. Todd was thinking "What is this going to cost us?" Little did he know how serious it was.

Todd says he parked as far away from the emergency room as humanly possible. The longer he walked, the more his thoughts began to race and consider the possibilities of what happened to me. As he got close to the entrance, he was met by a woman with a hospital ID badge. She asked if he was there for me and when he answered yes she quickly ushered him into an empty, private waiting room. She said the doctor would be in with an update soon. The only other thing she said was that I may have some bleeding in my head and they had already called the on-call neurosurgeon. Todd says he was in disbelief. I was 26 and healthy. He didn't understand what was happening.

Finally the hospital worker and a neurosurgeon came in. Todd says the doctor informed him as directly as possible that I had suffered a ruptured aneurysm, specifically a grade 4 or 5 subarachnoid hemorrhage. He asked how serious this was. She said major. He asked how major? She responded that my chances were 50/50.

Todd's mind was racing. How could this have happened? We had only been married 9 months. The doctor suggested Todd work on getting my parents here ASAP. She said time was not on our side. The doctor then led Todd to see me but she warned him I was still being worked on. He says what he saw was unimaginable. I was unconscious and had more tubes and wires connected to me than he thought possible. I was in critical condition on a respirator and surrounded by doctors and nurses. They were inducing me into a coma to let my brain settle down more easily. The doctors were thinking this would slow the blood flow to my brain meaning less bleeding.

Todd had the unenviable task of calling my parents and his family. He didn't have the number for my parents so a hospital representative helped him find it. He doesn't remember exactly what he told them-he just said they needed to be here. His Dad Raymond "Daddy O" lived about 30 minutes north of us but was in Chicago celebrating his birthday with family, which incidentally was the same day I collapsed. There was a party for him at my sister-in-laws house. She heard the phone ring and she says under normal circumstances she wouldn't have answered but something compelled her to. Todd told her what happened and she says the focus of the party shifted. They were concerned with getting Daddy O back to Florida as soon as possible.

Doctors told Todd that for the first 24 hours I would literally be fighting for my life. They had done all they could do to settle my brain. It was completely up to me now. Todd was only able to visit with me for a few minutes each hour.. He came in at 1 am and sat next to me, talking to me and holding my hand, He asked if I could hear his voice. I gently squeezed his hand. He wasn't sure if it was a twitch or if I was truly responding to him so he squeezed my hand twice. I then squeezed his hand twice. Todd says it was at that moment he knew I was going to survive. I don't remember doing that.

My parents couldn't get a flight to Ft Myers from Bowling Green, Kentucky until the next day. They were met at the airport by someone from the station who whisked them off to the hospital. Because I was in intensive care they were only allowed 20 minute visits every four hours. When my father-in-law arrived he came with a dozen roses in hand. But the roses couldn't stay in the room with me. So each time my family was allowed in, they brought the roses. I was conscious but my short term memory disappeared., so each time they came in I thought I was getting new roses!

I had several CAT scans, MRI's, and even an angiogram. Finally, after about a week they were able to determine I had bleeding near my brainstem from a ruptured brain aneurysm. . By this time I had a neurosurgeon Dr George Sypert, who said it was a delicate surgery, because the slightest nick or wrong move could mean bad consequences.

I ended up slipping into a coma for a period of time, which may have actually been a good thing. I was quiet. At one point, one of the many doctors tending to me told Todd he had never seen someone survive with as low of brain function that I had.

Todd says during his visit the next morning he remembers I recognized him. I was able to respond to his questions with head nods. But he was reminded several times by doctors I was not out of the woods yet. Even though I was acknowledging him I was facing an uphill battle. Days passed and I steadily showed progress. I was more alert and able to respond to people.

It wasn't until the 11th day after I was admitted that I was stable enough to undergo surgery. The doctor who performed the surgery likes to say he was operating on a swollen, angry brain, which is a great description. I had a number of stitches too many to remember exactly. I wasn't aware I even needed surgery. This time is very hazy for me and I honestly think that its for the best. My neurosurgeon said in his 25 years of operating on aneurysms he had never had one located so close to the brainstem. A lot of bodily functions are controlled by the brainstem so that's why it was so serious.

CHAPTER 2

Healing begins

Although I don't have any recollection of needing or having surgery I do remember soon after I woke up I hurt bad. I also couldn't lift my neck because muscles had been cut. I still wasn't sure what happened or where I was until I saw my Dad standing over me. He said "You're in the hospital. You had an aneurysm". I remember thinking Ok-then I was out again.

I lost some days after that but I remember thinking "What the heck is an aneurysm?" I had never heard of that before. I had to have someone explain to me that its basically a bubble on a blood vessel. Sometimes they're discovered before they burst but sometimes not. The cases of aneurysm rupture like mine are often deadly. My doctor says mine was a grade 5 subarachnoid hemorrhage. A subarachnoid hemorrhage is bleeding into the space surrounding the brain. Grade 5 being the worst. Thank God he was able to perform microscopic surgery in my brain to stop the bleeding. He placed a small metal clip on the blood vessel that had burst.

Now about God in all of this. I grew up with no religious background. I never went to church as a kid. I would spend the night with friends and go with them every once in a while. I didn't really even understand much about God. In fact, before Todd and I got married I was baptized in his church because I had never been baptized as a baby. I will say this-I had many people praying for me among them friends and family. Now that I look back I do believe their prayers did some good.

Because I was intubated I couldn't talk so I had to write everything down. My husband still has some notes I wrote while recovering from that surgery. They are actually funny. At one point I wrote "I have some friends coming over who will want/need oxygen" At first my handwriting was illegible, but I penned plenty of scribbles while trying to communicate. One day I asked my father-in-law where my mother-in-law was (she had died a few years earlier). Daddy O became flustered because he didn't want to upset me. He asked a nurse what he should say and she said tell her the truth. So Daddy O said his wife had passed away two years earlier from breast cancer. He says my eyes got as big as saucers and I put pen to paper writing for a long time. My message said "Then who have I been spending all this time with?"That brings chills to my spine today.

I spent most of my time in the critical care unit. My mom says they arrived one day and saw my hands tied to the bed. The nurse explained she had found me on the floor trying to get to the bathroom. I was so weak I didn't realize I couldn't walk. I also ran the risk of having vasospasms which are when blood vessels narrow limiting blood flow to the brain. Not good. I was in the ICU because of that risk and because it was protocol to be there after brain surgery.

Once I was stabilized it was soon time for me to leave that hospital and go to a different one for rehab. The nurses had all gotten together and bought me a gown, robe, and slippers! My family and I were very grateful and touched by their kindness. One of the nurses put her arm around my mom And said "You don't realize, in this unit, very seldom do our patients live". My mom says the tears flowed after that.

Now the hard work was beginning. I was starting physical therapy. That time is still a little hazy. I remember at one point waking up looking directly at my Mom and asking if she knew where my parents were. That had to just be heart-breaking for her. I haven't addressed that with her since then though because I don't want to bring up those emotions for her again.

It was a sign things weren't going well. I remember my husband and parents being in the room and they started talking about our wedding. I innocently asked "who's wedding?"They said yours. I was aghast-I wasn't married! Why were they saying that? I asked them and they reminded me we had gotten married the previous October. I still didn't believe them. If I was married, where was my ring? The hospital had taken all my jewelry so I had no proof. I recognized Todd; I just didn't realize he was my husband. I thought maybe we were boyfriend-girlfriend; but I had no idea he was my husband. Those memories of our wedding eventually came back though over a few weeks.

Being the news junkie I am, CNN was constantly on in my room. One time when my parents entered for their 20 minute visit I asked where Jodi was. My parents and Todd looked at each other and said they didn't know her. I said yes they did she was my roommate. My parents and Todd said I didn't have a roommate. I became adamant and said Jodi was my roommate at The Citadel. There was big news at that time that a woman had been admitted to the Citadel. My mom says that convinced her I was partially understanding the news.

But that was the beginning of a downhill spiral. I was doing poorly, having double vision, major cognitive problems and blinding headaches. My eyes were actually working independently of one another so I had to wear a patch on one. I had some fun and started talking like a pirate! But doctors and my parents were concerned. They did CAT scans and MRI's and determined one of the ventricles in my brain stopped working causing a buildup of spinal fluid. So it was back to the OR for me so doctors could insert a shunt in my brain to drain the fluid. Brain surgery number 2 therefore happened within a matter of weeks.

My sisters-in-law Rae Kyriazis and Lori Sandquist decided they needed to come down from Chicago to support Todd. Lori says she was not prepared to see me like she did. Me, a news anchor and reporter silenced, semi-conscious and still, almost peaceful in a chaotic way. She says they talked to me about everything and nothing, holding my hand, letting me feel their warmth. They were only allowed a 15 minute visit every few hours. As Lori says it was not enough time.

Lori went back to our apartment with Todd to take care of the dog and she noticed a pile of unopened mail on the table. Bills, bank statements, wedding invitations, magazines and other stuff. Suddenly, none of that mattered now.

CHAPTER 3

Not eating

I guess the effect of the shunt was remarkable. I recognized people again. I became aware that I was in the hospital and started asking questions. But it was hard to talk. I could only whisper because the bleed had paralyzed a vocal cord. I did have a tube in my nose that was used to feed me but I hated it. I hated it so much I kept pulling it out. I distinctly remember feeling something in my nose-then I started pulling and pulling. It was gagging me but I couldn't stop. I did that at least twice before doctors had enough. Daddy O remembers the day he walked into my room and saw I had pulled it out. It was a big old nasty mess! He quickly got the nurses who ran in and fixed me up.

Because I pulled out the tube at least twice, I ended up having what's called a PEG (percutaneous endoscopic gastrostomy) tube implanted in my stomach. That was the third surgery within a matter of weeks. I literally had a tube protruding from my stomach. During meals, nurses would come in and hook me up to what looked like chocolate milk. It worked because I wouldn't be hungry anymore. The only problem was the doctor ordered more than I could handle. I would tell the nurse I was getting full and she would say we have to give you all of it-doctors orders. After the third time of throwing up immediately afterward they decided I was right, it WAS too much. So they decreased the serving and all was good. I missed eating food but I had more important things to worry about.

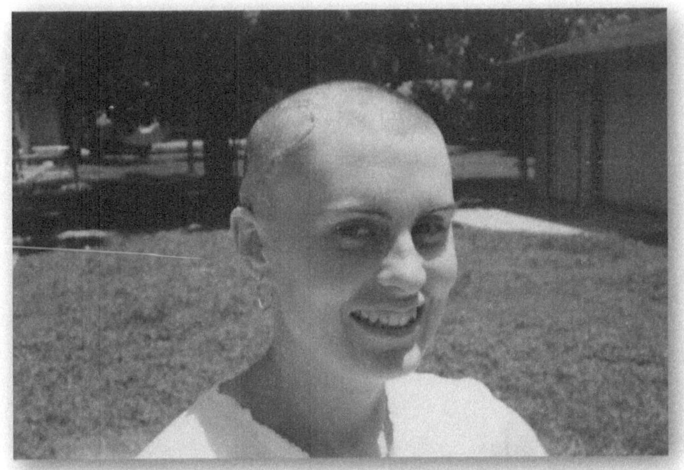

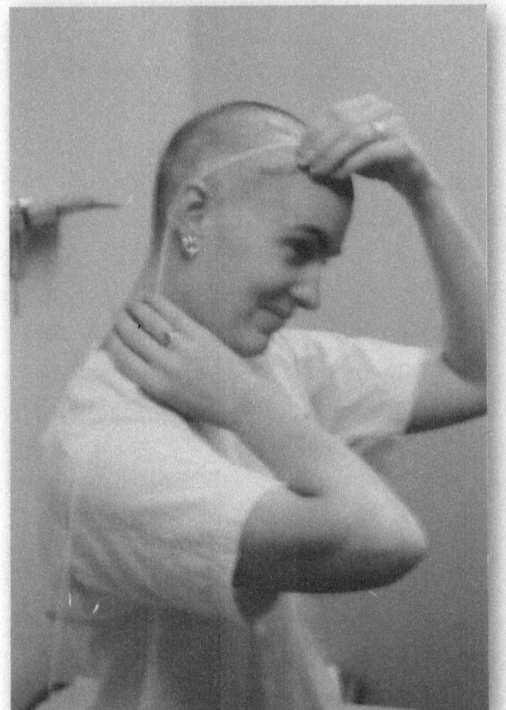

This is what my shunt looks like and where it goes.

CHAPTER 4

The real work begins

After I recovered from the PEG tube surgery I was transported back to the hospital I was previously in-this hospital specialized in rehabilitation. My days were spent in speech, occupational, and physical therapies. I'd eat breakfast about 8-start therapies at 9, have a break from 12-1, then be back at it until about 4 in the afternoon. It was good-I actually liked it because I had great therapists. I was a little confused about speech therapy-I thought I was having it because of my paralyzed vocal cord. In reality it was about communication skills. My therapist would show me pictures of objects such as a dog, A ball, and a pen and I would have to name them. Lucky for me I got them right. It didn't seem like work at all. Occupational therapy was more daily living activities-making sure I got the correct change if I went shopping for example. We also did some work in the kitchen preparing small meals. Physical therapy was just that-getting me stronger so I could walk unassisted again. I was in a wheelchair for a while, then a walker, then two canes, then I was discharged with one cane.

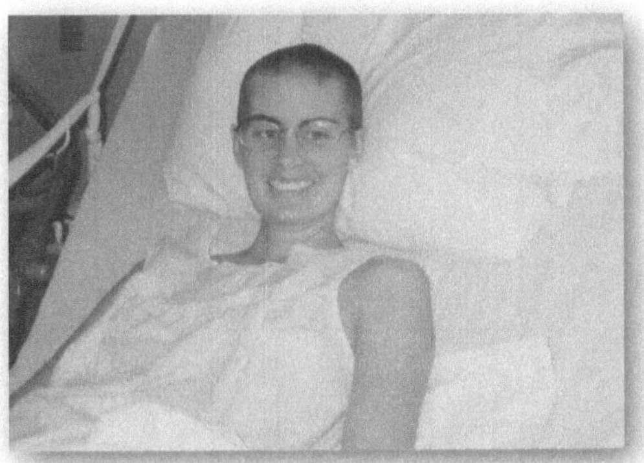

Me about a month into my hospital stay

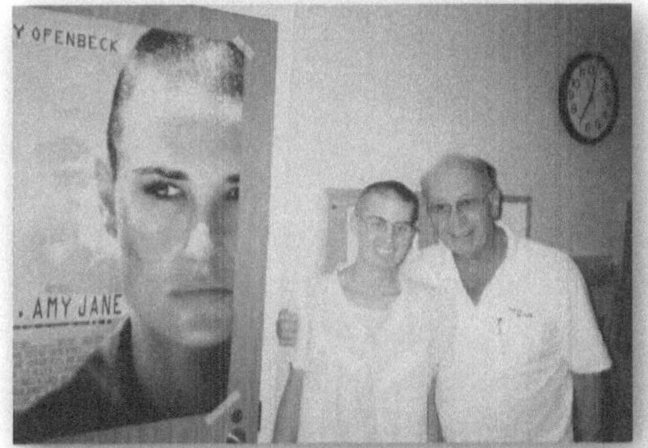

Demi Moore's movie GI Jane had just come out and a lot of people thought we looked alike bald. So Todd was able to get a movie poster and doctor it. My middle name is Jane so it was perfect. Todd wrote Demi Moore a letter and I ended up getting an autographed picture of her. My father in law is pictured with me.

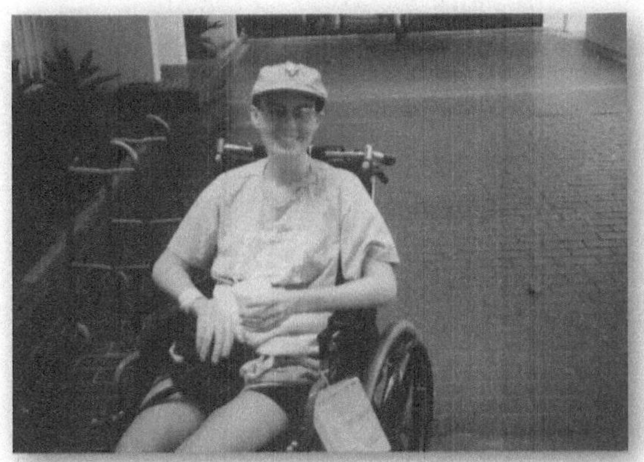

It was good to get out in the fresh air.

CHAPTER 5

Man's Best Friend

Things were going well. My hair was starting to grow back thank God! I've been told I looked good bald, but with all the scars and indentations on my head I was afraid that wasn't so. Hats were my friend for quite a while. I had visitors a lot which was nice. Probably the nicest thing was my father in law "Daddy O" was at the hospital all day every day with me shortly after I was admitted. He lived about 40 minutes north of us so it really wasn't any trouble. And boy did he watch out for me! He didn't hesitate to question the doctors or nurses if he thought something wasn't right.

As a thank you for coming to visit me I promised Daddy O I would take him to Hooters to lunch when I got out of the hospital. That soon became a standing lunch date. Daddy O would come to Ft Myers every week and we'd go to lunch somewhere new. Since I wasn't driving yet it was great.

Before we moved to Florida I worked at WSIL TV in Southern Illinois as the main anchor and reporter. We had been gone from there less than a year so when the station heard what happened to me they ran a story about me on the news. The reaction from viewers was simply amazing. I received hundreds of cards from people I didn't know. They had simply watched me on TV. That was so incredible to me and it was inspiring. I had people I didn't even know pulling for me, rooting for me to get better. It was a confidence builder. I still have all those cards and occasionally will pull them out and read them.

I was doing better, but I really missed my dogs. I had two, a lab chow girl named Bill (yes, a girl named Bill) and a German Shepherd female named Chase. I have to explain Bill-my husband is a trumpet player and his favorite musician is Bill Chase. He said when he got a dog he was naming it Bill no matter what. A friend found this dog wandering her street and called Todd. Of course he went over to see it and fell in love. Her brought her home and called her Bill. I tried to talk him out of it to no avail. So Bill it was. When we decided to get a German Sheppard, we knew she was going to be named Chase. Hence Bill and Chase.

I knew dogs were allowed in the hospital because I had visits from the therapy dogs there. So my husband asked if there would be any way I could have a visit from my dog. The hospital staff agreed it would be Ok, but I would have to go sit outside and visit. That was great! I was so excited and happy to see Bill. She was all soft and fluffy and she seemed excited to seem me. That really made my day. It was only one visit I got with her but it was the best and really did a lot for my mental health.

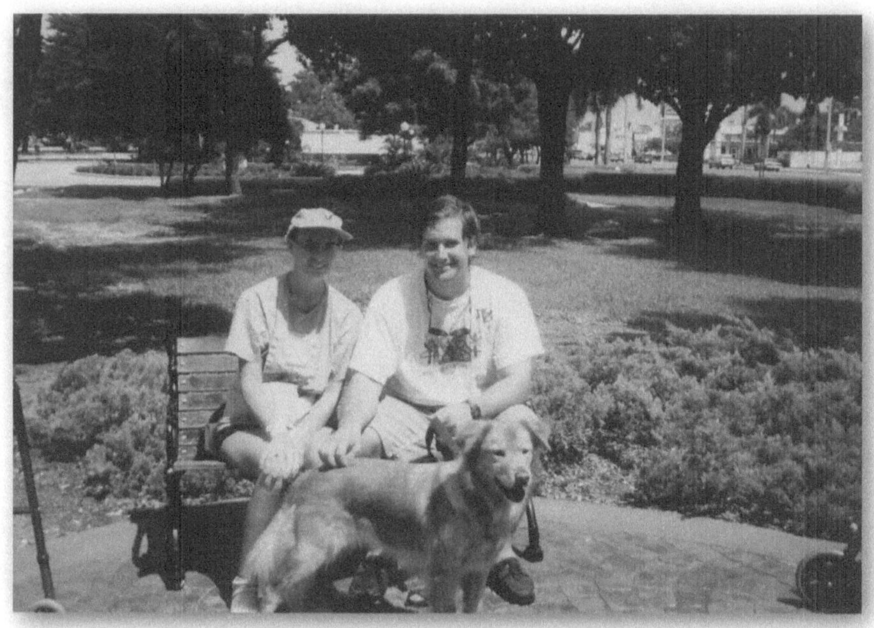

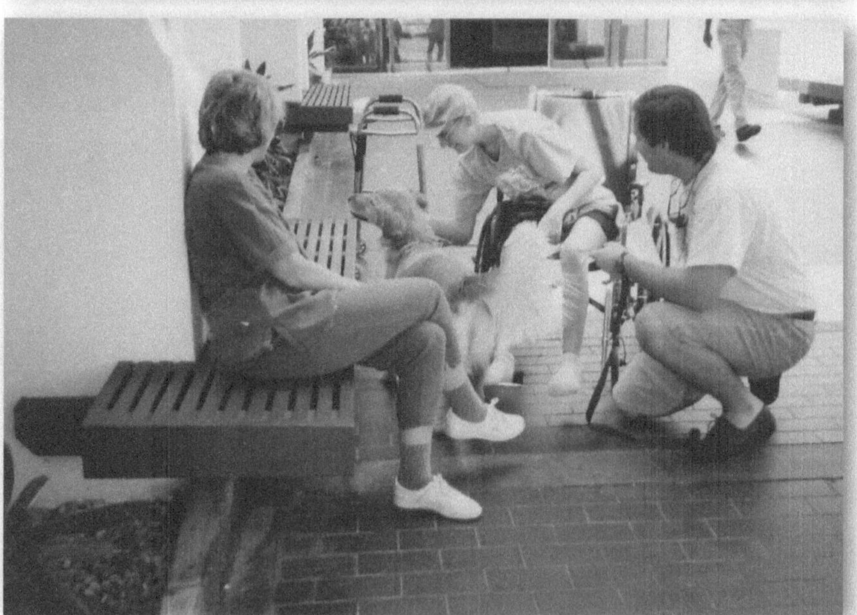

Todd and I and Bill the female dog. I was so happy to get to see her!!

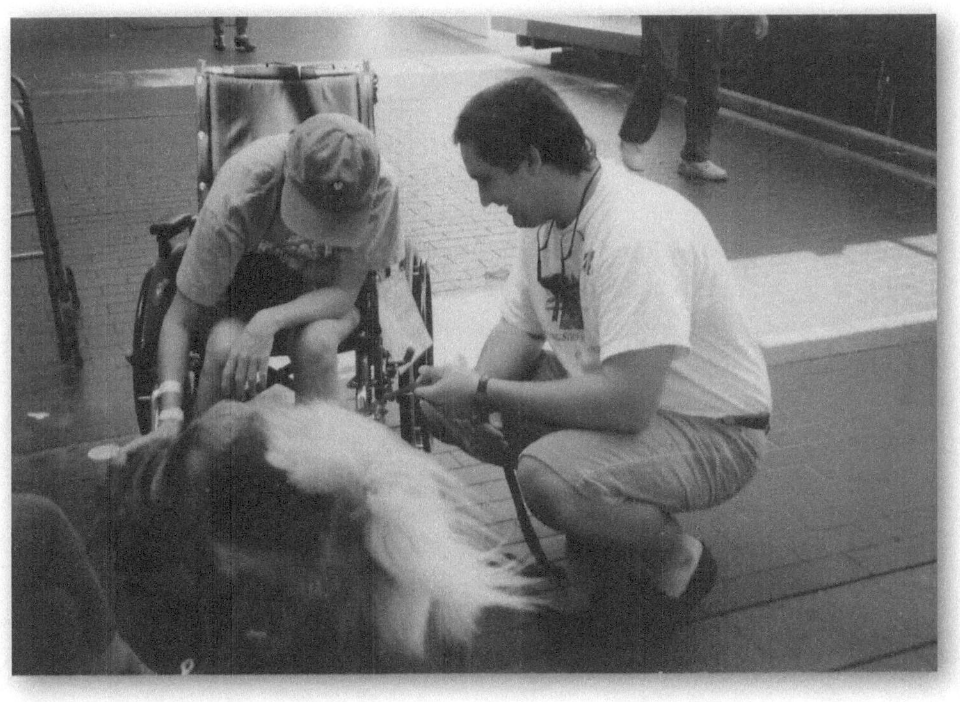

CHAPTER 6

I'm hungry

My goal was to eventually return to the job I loved so much. That is really what kept me going. I was IV free but I still had that annoying PEG tube in my stomach. I was beginning to learn again how to eat. I started with liquids-soups and juice. I remember a nurse there telling me to swallow deliberately and pronounced to be sure the food went in my stomach and not in my lungs. That could happen because my vocal cord was paralyzed meaning it couldn't close completely when I was eating. I then graduated to pureed foods. I didn't know what I was eating but it sure was good. I had several tests where I swallowed this thick liquid that was sickeningly sweet. Technicians basically took a live x-ray to make sure it was going into my stomach. Luckily it was.

I ended up spending my 27th birthday, August 31, in the hospital which was fine. I received balloons and flowers from family and friends. The nurses were all great even singing happy birthday to me during one therapy session! I really didn't mind being in the hospital that day. It was comfortable.

CHAPTER 7

Going home

I was progressing well. We spoke with my doctor about discharge and he suggested I continue outpatient physical, occupational, and speech therapies for as long as I needed them. I was going home. And it was appropriate they were discharging me on September 23 because that was my husband's birthday! What a birthday gift to both of us! My mom had arrived from Kentucky and was going to stay for a while to help. She drove me home and it was so exciting. I remember seeing things and recognizing them on the way home which was good news.

We got to my apartment, opened the door and I was greeted by two very happy dogs. The place was also inundated with balloons! My husband was at work but had gotten a bunch of them to welcome me home. It was good to be home but I was exhausted. I immediately went and laid down for about an hour. My husband came home from work very happy to see me there.

I had a few days off before I started outpatient therapies. Unfortunately, I still had that *&$#@%^ PEG tube in my stomach. It was clipped off but it was hanging at my waistline. It was challenging to shower and get dressed with it. It would be coming out soon via same-day surgery and I couldn't wait. This is gross but sometimes the clip would get loose or come off and my stomach juices would come spilling out. It was disturbing and inconvenient. I was counting down the days until it would be removed.

CHAPTER 8

The work continues

My first day at outpatient therapy arrived. I couldn't drive yet so I needed a disabled transportation service to take me. I was thankful for it. I would do speech therapy first, then occupational, then physical, so it was from 9 am until noon three days a week.

I continued what should be called communication therapy.. How to ask for help while in public, identifying certain objects, and stuff like that. I don't think I really had too much trouble doing the exercises, but there were a few that stumped me. I absolutely loved my speech therapist. She was so nice and encouraging. I would get flustered at times but she had a way of calming me down and supporting me.

I did different exercises in physical therapy to build my strength so I could get rid of the cane. I rode the air bike and lifted weights. I love to work out so that was fun. I also worked on my balance and did things like going up stairs. These were activities I had taken for granted. There was still a lot I wasn't able to do. I was using a cane to get around for one thing because my balance was still off and I was weak.

Occupational therapy was more for fine motor skills. There was a little peg board and I would put the pegs in the holes. It also dealt with daily living skills. I remember having to make macaroni and cheese one day in the kitchen. Again. I had great therapists so it was fun. I had a sense of gratitude for my life that until that afternoon in the gym had been missing. I then realized I had taken the simplest tasks for granted.

I spent about three months going through these various therapies and I was told I made remarkable progress. My goal was to get stronger and get rid of that cane! It made me feel old and like a gimp. I was a gimp but I didn't want to be anymore. The day it was taken away was a little nerve wracking but I was up to the challenge. I was definitely stronger and more stable so it was time. Now if my hair would hurry up and grow back I'd be happy!

Meanwhile my sisters-in-law decided they wanted to bring their families here for Christmas. Rae remembers Todd and I at Daddy O's-me with a new hat covering the hair that was starting to grow back. She vividly remembers watching me struggle with every little thing I did from walking to talking to eating. Everything had to be done deliberately and slowly. That night when we opened gifts they saved the best for last. They had gotten me an engraved plaque from "The O Team" that recognized me for my unrelenting fortitude and courage. I was very grateful for that and touched but I didn't think I was doing anything special.

CHAPTER 8

My voice

Therapy ended but my work didn't. I continued to work out at the gym at our apartment complex. I'm a fitness fanatic. I love to work out so it was no bother. Some people have asked if I was afraid to go back into the gym since that's where I collapsed. My answer is no, not at all. I knew the aneurysm wasn't really related to being at the gym. I knew I didn't have another one so I was confident I was safe to work out. The only other aggravating thing was my voice. I was still basically whispering. I'd be at a restaurant and get the obligatory "Oh you've lost your voice" comment. After about the fifth time of explaining no I had a paralyzed vocal cord, I just nodded in agreement.

I saw a voice doctor who suggested injecting Teflon in the paralyzed vocal cord to help restore my voice. We did a lot of research and discovered Teflon is temporary and mainly used in older patients. I needed my voice restored to broadcast quality so Todd and I scoured the Internet and discovered the Vanderbilt Voice Center in Nashville. That was perfect because Nashville was about an hour outside of Bowling Green Kentucky where my parents lived. So we would be able to just stay with them.

I contacted Vanderbilt and made an appointment. It was several weeks before I could get in but the day finally arrived. We flew up there the night before. The next day we walked in the office and the walls were lined with gold records from all the music stars they've treated! You name a country music artist and he or she has probably been there. That gave me a good feeling. My doctor was Dr Mark Courey and he was great. He did all kinds of tests and exams before giving me his prognosis. He explained he would make a cut in my throat right above the creases in my neck, go in and place an implant in the paralyzed vocal cord.

I would be semi-awake for the surgery because I would have to talk to them to be sure it was in the right place. Todd and I had a really good feeling about Dr Courey and scheduled the surgery. I waited roughly 10 months because it was recommended to wait that long. There was a chance the cord could start working again which is why we waited.

The day of the surgery I wasn't nervous, just anxious. I vaguely remember talking to them during the surgery-they had me sing the alphabet. I was awake enough to do that but I couldn't really feel anything which was good. My doctor said they asked me to sing and I asked if this surgery was going to make me a singer because I wasn't before. That brought a smile to my surgeon's face!

The days after the surgery were interesting. I had a drain hanging from my throat which was kind of creepy to me. I spent about three days in the hospital. My throat was sore and my voice raspy but I had a voice! My doctor said it would get worse before it got better and it did. We flew back home to Florida a few days after the surgery with instructions to be careful. Interestingly my doctor said I should avoid clearing my throat if at all possible.

I was thrilled I had a voice again! It was good enough that it was time to think about heading back to work.

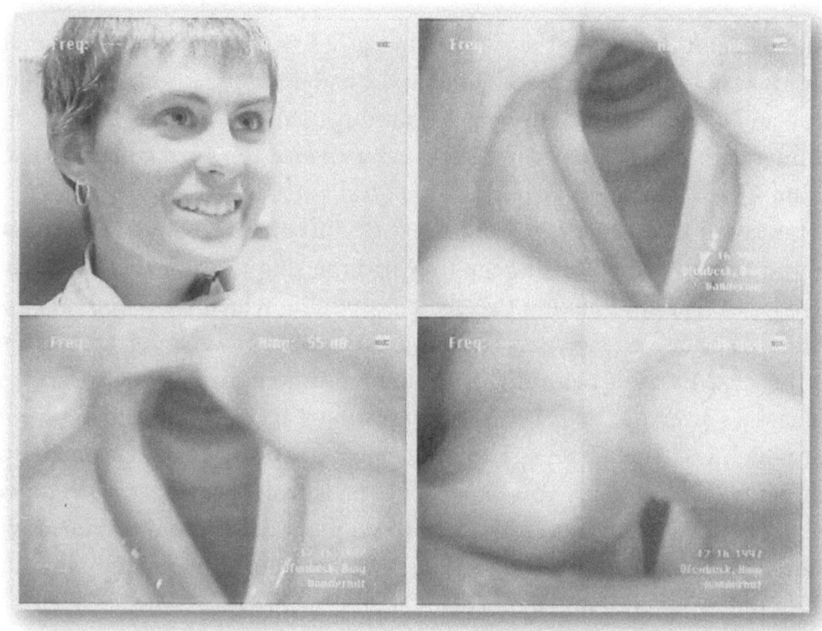

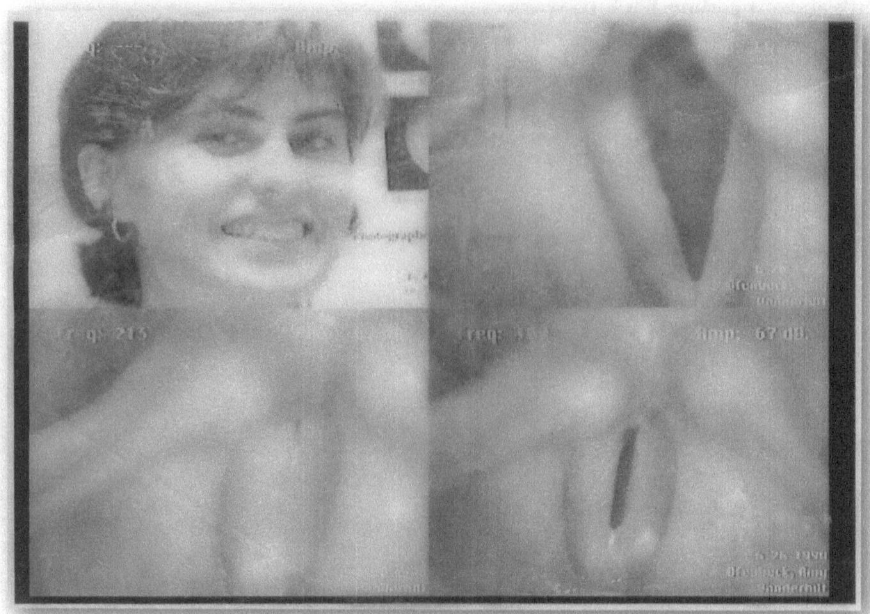

These are pictures of my vocal cords

CHAPTER 9

Going back to work

Nine months after the ruptured aneurysm I met with the news director at my station and told him I was ready to come back to work. However, I would need to start slow, working 2 days a week then gradually going back to full time. He agreed so we set a start date. I was so excited! I was ready to jump back in where I left off! Little did I know I was basically starting from the beginning, as if I had never done the job before.

My first day back was a day to get reacquainted with the staff and just the work in general. Most stations have morning and afternoon meetings where the staff is expected to present ideas for news stories for the day. I went to the morning meeting thinking I was just observing and getting back in the groove. I was surprised when they called on me for story ideas. I just said "Uh...what?" They explained to me that everybody had to have two story ideas every day ready to present. This was new to me. I didn't remember ever having to do that before. I was a little irked no one had told me ahead of time and just expected me to know that.

That was a sign of things to come.

I was a morning anchor and reporter before the bleed. I really wanted to get back on the anchor desk and actually practiced a few times. I was a better anchor than reporter. .I should mention that when I went back I started at the bottom working the worst shifts. I worked nights on weekends which in the TV news business meant I was there 2:30-11:30 pm Saturday, Sunday, Wednesday, Thursday, and Friday. Working nights during the week wasn't bad because there was always breaking news.

But I wanted back on a weekday day shift so I could spend more time with Todd and other friends who had normal work schedules. The assistant news director at that time knew that and was trying to make it happen. I have to say he was great to me. He really helped me and I could tell he wanted me to succeed. I got down and frustrated a couple times and he was always there to pick me back up. But a lot of my other co-workers were new and didn't understand my situation. Some of the producers also questioned me a lot about my stories and I would sometimes get irked looks from other reporters there when I was pitching my ideas.

As time went on, I eventually moved to a coveted day shift Monday through Friday. I was struggling coming up with story ideas though and got yelled at once for not having them. I honestly think this was due to the aneurysm. Before the bleed I could do just about any story I wanted because of the shift I worked. Plenty of times they were featured oriented or people related stories. Now I needed to do "hard" news which was just foreign to me. I put it in gear though working hard and was coming up with some. In the business, whoever has the idea reports and writes the story. But I found that if management liked my ideas they gave them to someone else. I really wasn't sure why but I'd still willingly hand over my notes. Often times I was left with nothing to do which was aggravating and boring. I was getting frustrated but I hung in there.

After a few months it got better but I wanted back on the anchor desk. There happened to be a weekend anchor opening on the ABC affiliate, which was the station I worked for. The management was holding auditions for the job. I was excited. I auditioned like everyone else and was told I was great. I felt good about it and was comfortable up there.

But it was not meant to be. I was passed over for the job and was disappointed. I saw it as a challenge though. I was determined to prove myself.

But my health was about to be a bigger challenge.

My husband and I were home one evening when I sneezed and felt like my head was going to explode. I had a sharp blinding pain in my head and my neck immediately stiffened up. This was in May 1999, not even two years after my rupture.

We called my neurosurgeon who ordered MRI's. The news was not good. My shunt was malfunctioning, causing spinal fluid to build up on my brain. Doctors needed to go in and fix it, which meant another haircut for me. I was most upset about losing my hair again because I was on TV-a bald reporter isn't exactly appealing for viewers.

I was admitted to the hospital on a Thursday morning and was home by Friday evening. Nothing like having brain surgery one day then being released the next.

CHAPTER 10

More bad news

I went back to work a few weeks later but I still wasn't feeling all that great. Because my head was shaved I needed a wig this time around for work. Todd and I went wig shopping and found a great one that was very similar to my hair. I wasn't nervous about it at all. I figured people at work would know and that was fine.

But I was still having pain. The shunt revision had been a month before and I just felt bad. My head was killing me and my neck was stiff and I was lethargic.

I went back to my neurosurgeon who ordered an MRI. The news would not be good. The shunt still wasn't working properly, so he needed to go in and figure out why. He couldn't really explain why this was happening. He just said shunts were unpredictable. All the research I was doing indicated he was right. I was preparing for him to have to replace the whole thing.

I had the surgery, The fourth brain surgery and the second within two months. My doctor said he replaced the shunt with a larger, thicker tube. He only had to replace the upper portion in my brain. Amazingly I was out of the hospital the next day! I had heard the term drive through surgeries which means short hospital stays-but drive through BRAIN surgery? The doctor said he was concerned about possible hemorrhaging in the brain but luckily that never happened. This was July of 1999.

I took about two weeks off work and even though I wasn't feeling great I went back to the station. The wig sure was getting good use. It was getting more difficult for me to go back and start over yet again. But I wasn't giving up yet. The normal eight-plus hour workday was exhausting but I really wanted to continue to try. If anything I'm perseverant and not a quitter.

CHAPTER 11

Back to the hospital

I was completely exhausted after work every day but I still plugged away. But not a month after the last surgery I was back in the operating room.

I had been at home after work one day when I sneezed again and again felt like my head was going to explode. It hurt severely, like nothing I had ever felt before.

It turned out the shunt still wasn't working. My right hand was also a little numb and weak which was a new symptom and a sign things were getting worse. So it was off to the hospital for brain surgery No. 5. At this point I didn't care. I was just feeling so bad all I wanted was for the pain to stop, and that meant more surgery. In your brain you have ventricles that collected spinal fluid and pump it throughout the body. One of my ventricles wasn't working again so spinal fluid was building up. The shunt was supposed to take care of that but it wasn't. Doctors went in and pulled the shunt back and it started working again. A few days after the surgery I was actually starting to feel better.

For some reason though my right hand was numb and weak so I was using a stress ball to strengthen it.

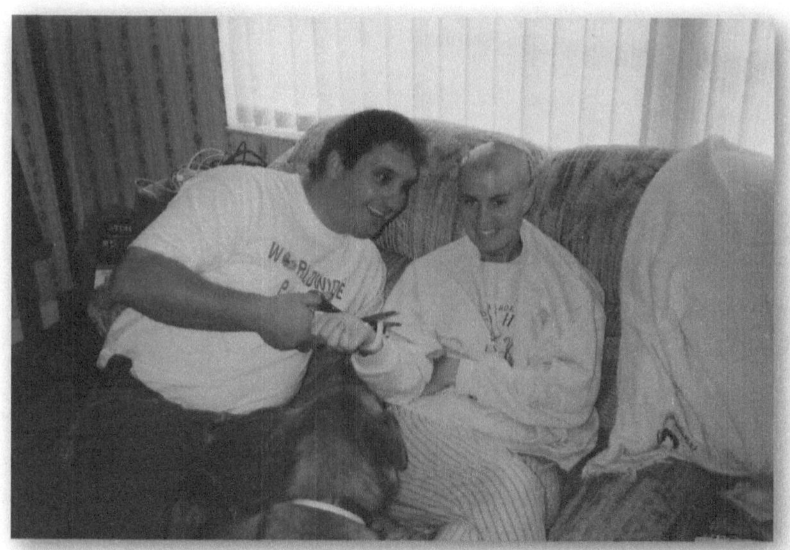

The cutting of the hospital bracelet! I'm free!

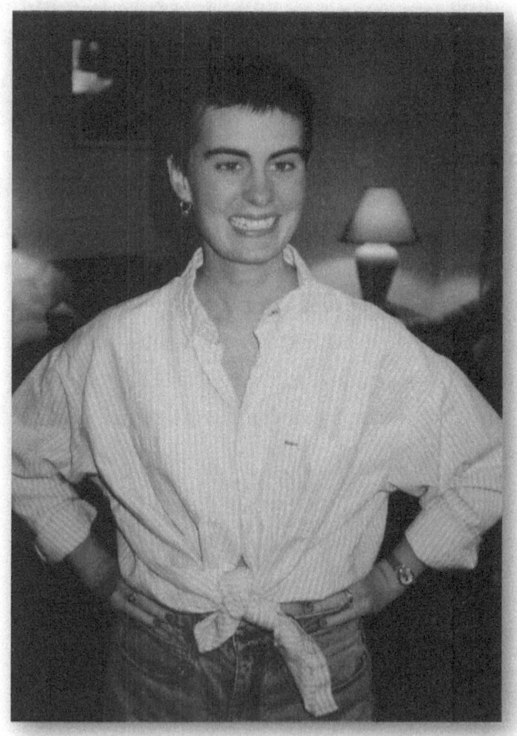

CHAPTER 12

Still feeling bad

Not even a month later, September of 1999, I was feeling awful and desperate. Desperate to find out why the previous surgeries weren't working. I was getting really discouraged too. It was just getting so hard to remain optimistic and positive. I didn't say anything to anybody though. I was trying to give the impression I was still positive and optimistic.

My doctor had the reputation of being one of the best neurosurgeons in the country and I trusted him. He suggested a procedure called a third ventriculostomy. That procedure meant he would cut a small hole in the thinned floor of the third ventricle, thereby draining the fluid. It's not the standard fix for hydrocephalus, but rather an alternative treatment.

I was willing to try anything. My doctor hadn't performed this surgery many times so he referred me to another associate in his practice who had. I had to wait a few weeks before I could have the surgery because the equipment had to come to Ft Myers from Tampa! My doctor was telling me he really needed to get inside my head and see what's going on. There was a chance the third vent wouldn't work, he said, and if that happened he would do what was called a stereotactic procedure, which meant he would use a 3-D system to locate a target and perform an action to alleviate the problem.

I was getting tired of having surgery but at the same time I was feeling awful and just wanted to feel better. I was over losing my hair. In fact, I was enjoying throwing on the wig and going. It took no time at all. The only problem was after wearing it for a few hours I started to get hot and itchy. I remember one of the first times I went back to the newsroom after six hours of wearing it I just wanted to get the thing off. I didn't care who saw me. I walked in to a crowded newsroom, ripped the thing off, and threw on a hat. The shock of my co-workers surprised me! I was sure everyone there knew I had a wig. Maybe they were just surprised by my nonchalance.

CHAPTER 13

Surgery #7

We scheduled the third ventriculostomy for March 2000. We talked with my doctor at length and we were confident in him and the procedure. It was going to be a long surgery about three hours. My other surgeries were about an hour. Regardless I had to do something because I was just feeling awful. This was brain surgery and haircut number 6. I wondered if I would have to leave the station because I just felt awful. I was growing tired of having to go back and start all over anyway.

Surgery day came. Much to our surprise, my doctor said he discovered a golf ball sized cyst pressing on the shunt causing it to malfunction. That's a pretty good sized cyst to have in your brain! The doctor punctured the cyst and the shunt started working again. My doctor said a cheer went up in the OR when that happened! It sounded like great news.

CHAPTER 14

My career is over

Two months later I made one of the toughest decisions in my life. I had to leave my job at the TV station. I was just struggling. There had been a lot of turnover and many of the new employees weren't aware of my situation. They became frustrated with me and didn't understand why I had trouble some days. I think they just decided I wasn't any good. My news director called me in one day and said it just wasn't working out. I was rather upset at the time. That was all I knew how to do-report the news. I reluctantly agreed to leave. During my exit interviews many of the managers and executives wanted to know when I'd be back. It broke my heart to say never because they too were disappointed. But eventually I did see it was for the best.

CHAPTER 15

A frightening time

Things in the meantime got messy and frightening. I was at home, looking for jobs when I started having delusional thoughts. One day my husband came home from work and asked me how my day was. I said well, so and so (a reporter) from the station came to visit. My husband was surprised to hear that because he had worked with her all day. He asked why just out of curiosity. I went into a detailed explanation about what I believed we talked about. But then I said the conversation turned bad and she started making fun of me. That totally alarmed Todd but he just listened and took notes.

He went to work the next day and asked the woman if she'd been over to see me. She said no of course. I'm not sure what my husband was thinking then, but I'm sure it confused and worried him. This went on for a few months. I kept telling my husband that I had talked to several people. It affected my job too. By this time I had a new job working at the front desk of the Wellness Center of Fort Myers. I was sure people were out to get me. I was sure I was about to get fired and often begged my husband to call my boss and talk to her. They knew each other so it wouldn't have been strange.

I should also note I wasn't taking my meds. I didn't feel sick why did I need them? I was perfectly fine. I didn't need any medicine. This was July of 2000.

I began writing all these thoughts and feelings down. It was cathartic for me and a release. The only problem was when I would go back and read them I became even more convinced they had happened. So it was a double edged sword. We still have them and I'm tempted to read them, but my husband doesn't think that would be a good idea. He's probably right.

I would sit at the computer for hours just typing away. The one thing I remember is I kept asking why no one believed me. This stuff happened, I swear. I can recall the smallest details. But why don't people believe me? It was so disheartening and really bringing me down.

Perhaps the most frightening thing happened one night while at home with my husband. I was refusing to take my meds and he was begging me to take them. I still said no. At one point I even threw the pills in the toilet.

But then I remember thinking he took a handful of pills and tried to shove them down my throat. That didn't happen but I could've sworn it did. I came to the conclusion that he had tried to kill me. I was thinking my parents took a life insurance policy out on me and he wanted to collect. I was beside myself and panicking. I decided I had to leave. I was tired of Todd not believing me when I was telling him things were happening. And now this? I had to go.

I was serious and started packing a bag. I was just going to go to a hotel and stay while I figured out what to do. My husband panicked. He somehow got me in the car and took me to the hospital. I remember going into the ER and just being hysterical. They took me back and then I don't remember what happened.

CHAPTER 16

Dr's orders

Next thing I know I'm in a hospital room. A very tall intimidating white haired guy in a suit came in. He said "Hi Amy I'm Dr Schaerf (pronounced sheriff)." I knew that was a lie and I told him so.

"You're not a dr," I said laughing.

He said "Then who am I?"

I said "You're a cop."

"Do you need to talk to a cop?" he asked.

I said yes because my husband tried to kill me. He asked how? I told him he tried to shove pills down my throat. He listened to my ramblings for a while and started me on some medication I decided I would take.

But I was a mess for a while. I recall one time when the doctor was coming in I stripped off my gown and was just lying naked on the bed. Or at least I think I did that. I have no idea what he said or why I did that but I'm pretty sure it happened. I was on the psych floor so I don't think my actions were too shocking or they surprised anyone. I remember not having any visitors. Not even my husband which in hindsight was for the best.

I spent about five days in the hospital but it seemed shorter than that. I gradually starting trusting Dr Schaerf and realized he was here to help. He asked me if I felt safe going home with Todd. Somehow I said yes. I was also thinking what choice do I have? I have nowhere else to go. He kept asking me that question and I couldn't figure out why. He also kept asking me if I had any thoughts about harming myself. Of course not-why? I realize now he was obligated to ask me that in the event I did hurt myself. And I had forgotten what brought me to the hospital.

I went home with orders to see Dr Schaerf three times a week. I think my husband went to many of the appointments with me. I didn't really understand what was going on. I just told the doctor what I was feeling and what I thought was happening. Dr Schaerf says this is a classic case of someone who has had insults to the brain and now the chemicals in my brain were off. He says all the surgeries I have had disrupted the connections in my brain also. Medicine helps make me normal again. He says its similar to being a diabetic in that I will need medicine forever to keep me stable.

I ended up starting a pretty powerful antipsychotic medication called Zyprexa that unfortunately caused me to gain weight. That was the least of my worries however. I had to sort through these thoughts and I really wanted to understand why this was happening. My diagnosis was organic affective disorder which really didn't mean anything to me. Dr Schaerf tried to explain to me that when that large cyst was removed from my brain it created a hole that my brain was now able to fill up. That just sounded so made up to me and I was resistant to that explanation at first. I have since learned organic affective disorder means a mood disorder brought on by a physical change.

I started getting better and more stable, mostly seeing physician assistants as I improved. An interesting note from Dr Schaerf-he says we create our own stigma by hiding. I was having trouble with the fact I would be on an anti-psychotic medicine for the rest of my life but Dr Schaerf says my illness is much like people with diabetes or depression or other chronic illnesses. And he says researchers are always introducing new medicines to the market so there are advances being made.

CHAPTER 17

Getting back to normal

I was ready to get on with things and start working again. I was scouring the internet and newspaper ads for jobs. I found a position was available at a retirement community golf course. It was perfect for me because I grew up playing golf and working in pro shops. I interviewed for the job and was thrilled to learn I got it. I started shortly thereafter and was completely overwhelmed by things. I couldn't remember how to work the cash register or how to sign people in. I had purposely not told my boss about my history because I didn't want to scare him off. But things were not going well. He ended up moving me from the pro shop and having me be a ranger out on the course. That meant I just made sure the foursomes were moving along and weren't holding others up. I hated it and often just went to a hole far away from the golf shop and parked my cart there for a while. I figured out I was of sight, out of mind.

One day about a month after I started the pro called me in. I knew he was going to fire me and in one way I was relieved because I was so miserable. When he said things weren't working out I came clean., I said I had had a number of brain surgeries and had some memory problems. Could he give me some extra time and help? His answer-no. I was a little surprised he didn't seem to care one bit. I left that day in tears. I was extremely disappointed he didn't want to help me. I wondered Is this the way it was going to be from now on? I went home and told Todd I had gotten fired. He comforted me as usual, thank God.

CHAPTER 18

A volunteer job

I live across the street from a major hospital and we worked out at a gym that was there so I had stuff to occupy my time. Plus I was doing pet therapy with my dog named Bill. I had such a positive experience when I was a patient I wanted to give back. So every Thursday I would take Bill to the hospital and we would visit the patients.

One day I happened to run into the public relations director for the hospital and we had a nice chat. I told her I wanted to get into public relations now; did she have any openings? She said no. I persisted though and asked her if I could shadow her for a few days just to get my feet wet. She said sure she'd love to have me. I became a volunteer in the public relations department three mornings a week.

I was really hoping to learn more about public relations and maybe even write some press releases and make media calls. But I did nothing like that. I ended up doing menial work like taking a ruler and measuring newspaper articles that just mentioned the hospital. I had no idea why and I don't even think I was doing it right. I thought the PR director wasn't using me to her advantage. I had contacts at TV stations and I knew what it takes to get media attention. I pressed her for more but all I got was a sympathetic smile.

CHAPTER 19

A good job

I continued to look for jobs while volunteering. I found a part time position at the medical library at the hospital. I had no experience but thought why not? I applied and ended up getting the job. I knew nothing about libraries though. I began training and was completely overwhelmed. It didn't help that my boss was very cold. She never smiled, never once asked me how I was. She barely trained me. I don't think I lasted two weeks there before she fired me. Fine by me. But still it was job number 3 within a matter of months.

I was beginning to see this as a challenge. I knew there had to be something out there for me. I continued working out at the gym to occupy my time. I was beginning to get to know everybody there from the trainers to the management so it was fun. I went in one day for my normal workout and the manager was very harried. I asked if everything was OK and she asked if I knew anyone looking for a job. I just about jumped over the counter screaming "Me! Me!" She explained she was looking for a front desk attendant-someone to greet gym-goers and do some cash register work. Was I interested? "You betcha!" I said.

I went through the proper steps and was thrilled when I got the job. I was a little more comfortable because I knew many of staff members and clients of the gym. I was working Monday through Thursday from 4-9 pm. Perfect because I could get in a workout before work and I had Fridays off. Again I didn't tell my new boss about my surgeries because I was afraid I'd scare her off. I just knew this job was going to be different.

CHAPTER 20

Rough first day

I started my first day at the gym and was completely overwhelmed of course. This job had to work out, it just had to. But not telling my boss my medical history was a mistake. It wasn't going well and not even a week on the job she called me in to tell me I was fired. I broke down and begged her to give me another chance and I told her my story. She said she knew about me from an article that was in the paper about me. I can't remember what came of that conversation but I left and went home.

My memory problems meant I didn't remember getting fired so I showed up for work the next day. She was completely surprised and said point blank I fired you yesterday. I again begged and pleaded for her to give me another chance. I asked for extra training and help with the promise if I couldn't do the job in a month I'd leave. She agreed.

It took about a month before I understood how to work the cash register and run the check in computer. I worked until closing which meant I had to reconcile the cash drawer and lock everything up. That cash drawer was my nemesis. I hated that thing. I do not like working with numbers so that didn't help. But I soon got the hang of it. I was told if I had any problems to give my boss a call at home which I did. She often talked me through it.

I was finally doing well. I was in the best shape of my life since I worked at a gym and I was beginning to come out of my shell. My job required I greet gym-goers and I was loving all the new people I was meeting.

CHAPTER 21

A new beginning

I worked at the gym four days a week and spent weekends at the beach with Todd and friends. It was great!

The delusions were still there sometimes. They'd come in spurts. One day I'd be great, the next I'd be a mess thinking these bad things were happening. I had a great boss at the gym and I ended up telling her everything. She was sympathetic and helped me through them. That job at the gym was a turning point for me. I became more confident and I was happy.

That all changed one day. There were rumors the gym was being sold to the hospital, but I hadn't heard anything official. Then one day I was called into my boss' office with the head trainer. They both informed me there were going to be some layoffs and unfortunately I and four others were a part of that. I was so devastated and just broke down right there. I begged and pleaded for my job, but because the hospital was buying it the workers there had to be hospital employees and I was not. I was devastated.

I went home and explained to my husband I was going to be out of work. He knew I wanted to work so he scoured the Internet and discovered I was able to use the Division of Vocational Rehab since I was on disability. I made an appointment and went in and discussed my options.

They said they needed to evaluate me and my abilities so I went in one day for various tests. I was there from 10 in the morning until 4:30 that afternoon taking various tests and filling out forms. That totally wore me out! We did a lot of memory work which was frustrating. It was interesting; my short term memory was bad, but give me about 15 minutes and it was fine! They would give me a list of ten words and I would have to repeat them. I would have to define words for them, I had to do some math, and I looked at pictures and picked out what was wrong in them. I remembered doing a lot of stuff like that when I was in the hospital.

It would be a few weeks before I would get the test results back and I was anxious. The day finally came and I was shocked to learn they estimated my IQ had dropped 15 points since before the aneurysm! That was really depressing and eye opening for me.

My interests and abilities were matched up with jobs. They said I matched with a reporter/correspondent position and recreation worker which were two jobs I have held in the past. They also said I scored high in the food preparation worker field and child care which totally shocked me because I don't like to cook or really be around kids. I'm not sure I believed that those jobs were matches.

In the meantime, I had decided I wanted off some of the medication I was on. I was taking an awful lot of them and I questioned whether I really needed them. The psychiatrist placed me on a med for attention deficit disorder and I guess it helped but I didn't think it was necessary to take it anymore. He also talked to us about me starting another memory med. I had been taking Aricept which is mainly for people with Alzheimer's. He said he had several patients who had experienced trauma and were taking a different Alzheimer's drug, but I wanted to get off the medication, not take more. So I decided against it. I was learning to live with my memory the way it was and I just did not want to add another medication to the mix.

CHAPTER 22

Goodwill calls

In early 2004, I was feeling the best I've ever felt. I was in great shape and loving life. Now if I could just find a job! The department of vocational rehab referred me to Goodwill, which I soon discovered was an employment service for the disabled. I had no idea they did that. I thought they were just a used clothing store. I met with the job counselor there and explained I wanted to go into public relations. That just seemed like a natural transition from news. I always thought when I was done on TV I would end up in public relations, I just never expected it to be so soon. The job counselor there suggested I volunteer in the public relations department there for a little bit. I didn't really want to. I knew I could do the job and I wanted to get paid. So I reluctantly agreed. I didn't have anything else to do.

I started and it was great. The women in the office were so nice and so willing to work with me. I was contacting the media, writing press releases, and getting them attention with all the contacts I had. I was feeling the best I ever felt. And to top it off, I found out they were creating a position for me. I had proven myself! I was told it would probably be a contract position, meaning they would evaluate it at the end of the year and see if it was worth it to bring me back. This was in July of 2004. So I basically had five months to prove myself. I could do it! I was up for the challenge and just so excited to be joining the workforce again.

CHAPTER 23

I can do this!

I found out I was selected to receive an award from the mayor of Ft Myers called the Mayor's Alliance award, which honors people with disabilities and their workplaces. I found out a Goodwill board member I had just met submitted my name which was such a nice surprise and a real honor. I was beginning to embrace the fact I was a disabled worker. I thought this could be a good, positive thing. I wanted other disabled people to know they too can be successful productive members of society with a little hard work. It was a real honor to receive that award. I was confident and happy again.

CHAPTER 24

Not Again

Not a month later I started feeling bad again. My right hand was feeling tingly and I just couldn't use it well. I saw my general practitioner who treated me for carpal tunnel syndrome. The meds didn't do anything though and when the headaches started I knew it was time to see my neurosurgeon again. I thought maybe it was my shunt malfunctioning, and I was practically an expert in this now.

But the problem was much more serious. I had a syrinx or cyst in my spinal cord the result of something called chiari (kee-are-ee) malformation. Chiari is a condition in which the cerebellum portion of the brain protrudes in the spinal canal causing a syrinx or cyst to form in my spine. Its been said that people with chiari have too much brain to contain which is very appropriate. It's a pretty serious thing that can result in paralysis so what choice did I have? I wasn't feeling great by any means. I needed to have yet another surgery to stop the progression of this disease.

We discussed this at length with my neurosurgeon Dr Gary Correnti. During this visit we looked at previous MRI's and we discovered the syrinx was starting to form then. But because I was having other issues it was overlooked. Dr Correnti says he spent a lot of time pouring over my recent scans looking for anything. Then he spotted something. He confirmed the diagnosis. But he hadn't performed the surgery very much and wanted me to see someone who had. To me that's the sign of a great doctor, when they refer you to someone else with more expertise. I was referred to Dr William Friedman at Shands Hospital which is at the University of Florida in Gainesville.

We drove five hours north to meet with him and he strongly suggested I have the decompression surgery. This development was a direct result of the aneurysm rupture and the trauma to my brain. Having decompression surgery meant the doctor would remove a small piece of my skull from the back of my head to help alleviate the pressure from the spinal fluid. I was resigned to the fact I needed yet another surgery. If I didn't have it, I would probably be paralyzed and I certainly didn't want that. We scheduled the decompression for Friday, December 3, 2004 in Gainesville. My parents would be making the trip from Kentucky for it. I was feeling bad so I just wanted the pain to go away. Little did I know it would only get worse.

I spent six days in the hospital for the decompression surgery. I remember getting discharged from the hospital with a walker because I could hardly move. I will never forget the five hour drive home. Every little bump we hit I screamed out in pain. My head and neck were just killing me. It was a horrible ride home and there was nothing my poor husband could do about it. I was also having trouble with my right side. It was numb and useless basically. I am right-handed and was then having to eat left-handed and I couldn't even hold a pen to write. I was really struggling and beginning to wonder why I even had the decompression surgery to begin with.

CHAPTER 25

Getting better

I could start physical and occupational therapy right away. I knew where I wanted to have it-I wanted it at the gym where I had worked. It was affiliated with the hospital now and I knew it would be good. When I went in for my initial consult I was barely moving using a walker to help me get around. The goal was to get me independent of any assistive devices no matter how long it took. I was prepared for it to be a while because I was just not good.

I spent five months going through physical therapy three times a week. When I started I was barely moving with a walker, then I used two canes, then one, then finally I was independent. I was moving slowly but I was moving on my own. My therapists said they've done all they can do for me-now it was up to me to maintain the strides. I remember asking one of my therapists if he thought I'd improved and his response was "Are you kidding me?! By leaps and bounds you've improved!" That made me feel good and was encouraging. Now it was time to go back to work. I was still in a bit of pain but was told it was normal.

CHAPTER 26

You Can Survive

I went back to work and basically picked up where I left off. I decided I wanted a new challenge though and sought a different job. I was able to get a job working for shop goodwill.com which is Goodwill's auction site like eBay. Our higher end donations such as designer clothes and jewelry get sent to us and we write item descriptions and list the items. It's great for me because I love to write.

The remaining issue now is pain. It's been about 11 years since the decompression surgery and I still hurt. Every morning I wake up because of pain. Head and neck pain can be so brutal and debilitating. Some days it gets better as the day goes on other days its excruciating all day long. I see a pain management doctor who is doing the best he can for me. I also have seen a chiropractor who uses lasers on me. Its just something I have to deal with. My husband seems to think I have a high tolerance for pain. Some days I'm just in tears because it hurts so bad. But I'm getting used to it and realizing that's just how its going to be.

My husband has some very kind words for me. He says I have more issues to deal with daily now than ever before. But my determination, fighting through my physical and psychological conditions every day and night inspire him in profound ways. He says the fact I pick myself up and try my best every day regardless of how bad I feel is a lesson everyone can learn from.

So that's where I am today. Relatively healthy and working and exercising. In some ways I can't believe everything I've been through. I don't know how I've been able to do so well. Some people have commented that I must be very strong but I say I'm not doing anything anyone else wouldn't do. I'm just trying to survive and live a happy productive life. I think I'm doing that for the most part. I still face health challenges every day, but I'm so used to it it doesn't faze me anymore. If there's anything I'd like people to take away from my story that is its to never give up. It may be tough sometimes, but you can survive. I did and so can you whatever your challenges in life may be.

Amy

By Craig Wolf Courtesy of the Island Sun newspaper Sanibel Island, Florida 2000

After more than two years of working with her, I'm saddened to say I really didn't get to know Amy Van Patten that well. And now that she's left our newsroom, the enormity of her story has hit me hard.

Many of you may know Amy. She came to our sister station, ABC 7, three years ago as a reporter and anchor with a promising future in broadcasting. An already skilled journalist and accomplished golfer, she had a winning way about her that was contagious...in a business that could use more sincere, smiling faces. With her husband Todd, a burly but friendly Desert Storm veteran and excellent photojournalist, this was a husband-and-wife team that would be an asset to any workplace.

Then 2 years ago this July, Amy's world came crashing down on her and her family. She suffered a brain aneurysm while working out at a local gym. 5 brain operations later, Amy just announced her most recent comeback attempt had taken too much of a toll on her. Not yet 30, Amy Van Patten is now on indefinite leave of absence from ABC 7. And the newsroom, shared with the staff at NBC 2 is a lesser place.

Through all of this, many of us were quick to comment how far Amy would've gone in television news. How unfortunate it was that this newspaper publisher's daughter who came to us from central Illinois missed several opportunities to move ahead at the station. How her great communication skills would never get to be fully utilized.

That's all changed now. Even in the transient world of TV news, even under the cynical watch of youthful but grizzled co-workers, and even in a pressure-cooker environment where you're best known by your most recent live shot....the Amy Van Patten story is now about one thing and one thing only: a beautiful young woman struggling to regain the health that most of us so take for granted.

Believe me, none of the above thoughts are meant to write Amy off. After seeing her for the past 2 years, bravely returning to work wearing the scar-covering wig that she was first to make fun of.....and continually going back for brain surgery after brain surgery...all with that incredible smile on her face....I am CONVINCED of this:

Amy Van Patten will be back.

Will To Live Trumps Odds-Denise Scott, The News Press December 13,2011

One minute on July 15,1997 Amy Van Patten was following her usual routine, lifting weights at the gym after leaving work for the day.

The next minute, the then 26 year old WZVN news reporter clutched her head and collapsed. An aneurysm had burst in her brain, taking with it her short term memory.

"I basically had no idea I had this ticking time bomb in my head." she says while resting at home two days before her sixth brain surgery. The most severe health problem on her medical record before this was asthma.

"I didn't have headaches," she says of the warning sign noting aneurysms are more common in older people. "I don't smoke. I was into healthy stuff. I went to the gym every day after work. Everything was great."

She had been married to her husband Todd Ofenbeck, who was 27 then, for just ten months. He also works for Waterman Broadcasting as assistant director of photojournalism. When he was called in from an assignment, he thought his wife had probably passed out from dehydration.

"Immediately a liaison sat me down and said "We don't know what's with her. She's unstable."Which was horrible. What do you mean? Why? Give me something."

Ofenbeck asked if he should call her parents. The liaison said yes. He had to sit in the hospital for close to an hour before he could see his wife.

During that time, he tried to focus on the positive. He thought about how lucky she was to have been in a public place.

"Where she works out a couple of nurses were there who knew what to do," he says. "She could've been driving, could've been home alone."

He told himself she was getting twice the expertise because she was brought in at shift change.

Then he saw her.

""She had tubes all over the place and was twitching uncontrollably," he recalls. "She was pale. Her eyes rolled back in her head. I talked to her and held her hand and cried on her to let her know I was there."

This couldn't be the end.

"The first night, they said she could come out fine, she could come out in a wheelchair...there were infinite possibilities," Ofenbeck says. "Anything I got from her at all was a blessing."

After drugs took effect to calm her body, Van Patten was moved into the critical care unit.

About 2 am, a nurse let Ofenbeck come in and sit by her side.

"She was sleeping soundly and I was talking to her," he says. "Finally she squeezed my hand and I knew everything was going to be all right."

Van Patten doesn't remember what happened to her that day or week preceding the hemorrhage. Her first memory is waking up in the hospital and seeing her husband and parents standing over her.

Flipping through a small yellow notepad, Ofenbeck says that was about four days after the aneurysm ruptured. The surgery to repair it happened nine days into her hospital stay.

"I kind of kept a diary when this whole thing started," he says, pointing to his scribblings of the liaison's name, the word aneurysm and 50/50-her chances of survival.

"Time kind of takes away some of the feelings", he says, looking at his notes. "How did she make it through this, especially alone the first night? Looking at the 50/50 gives you goose bumps".

Ofenbeck and Van Patten's parents weren't allowed to say in her room. They could only visit for 15 minutes every three hours.

"She would never remember any of them," he says of the visits. "So it was like seeing us for the first time every time."

At one point, she looked up at her mother and said, "Nancy do you know where my parents are?"

Time hasn't dulled the pain of remembering for Nancy Van Patten, who learned to read her daughters CAT scans during the ordeal. She speaks through tears three years later.

"Its amazing she made it through the aneurysm and everything else she's gone through," she says. "I don't know where she got her determination."

To brighten the mood at the hospital, Ofenbeck and the Van Pattens would bring the same flowers back into the room every visit.

"It was so funny because each time she thought she was getting new (ones)," her mother says.

Early on, Van Patten was disoriented and repetitive. After seeing a television show about The Citadel, she confused her own life and told stories about her experience as a cadet.

" I didn't remember I was married," she says, although she recognized Ofenbeck as her boyfriend. The hospital had removed her wedding ring, increasing her confusion.

Her husband joked with her parents he hoped she wouldn't come out of this with a newfound love of country music.

"Because of were the aneurysm happened and all the nerve endings at the base of the brain, the doctor said it was microscopic surgery to weave his way between all those nerves," Ofenbeck says. "If anything were damaged, it could affect anything-her ability to blink, to move..."

Dr. Jaime Alvarez, a neurosurgeon with Southwest Florida Neurosurgical Associates (The Sypert Institute) in Fort Myers and Cape Coral, performed Van Patten's most recent surgery. He says about half the people who suffer such massive brain hemorrhaging don't even make it to the emergency room. 'Her positive outlook on life has a lot to do with her recovery," he says.

While its uncommon for people as young as Van Patten to suffer from a brain aneurysm rupture Alvarez says it's not unheard of. Its more common between ages 50 and 70, with the exception of congenital aneurysms that can affect teenagers.

While the initial surgery took only about 45 minutes, Van Patten was out of Ofenbeck's sight for four hours, including pre-surgery preparation and recovery.

"Things go through your mind that no one at my age should be thinking about," he says of the wait. "I was 27 years old and potentially considering what to do with my wife as far as life support. The time, it seemed like days going by."

After the surgery, Van Patten was checked for responsiveness and given nerve tests. She couldn't life her head because neck muscles had been cut. They would heal with time.

But one of her vocal cords was paralyzed, turning her voice into a raspy whisper. With no gag reflex food could have gone into her lungs. She was fed by tube until rehabilitation trained her vocal cord to move again.

"I had to learn everything from eating to walking to writing," she says. "I fell flat on my face in critical care when I got up to try to go to the bathroom."

Spinal fluid began to build up in her brain, so a second surgery was done to install a shunt to drain it. Alvarez says the shunt is a catheter placed deep inside the brain., It attaches to a valve-which juts out as a small bump beneath the skin on the side of her head-and continues down into her abdominal cavity, where the fluid is absorbed.

She has since ad three "minor" surgeries, or revisions, to adjust the shunt and improve drainage. Alvarez says revisions are common because shunts, as man made objects, often clog and increase pressure.

"What tips me off to the shunt not working is horrible headaches and my neck gets really stiff," she says. A simple sneeze can cause the shunt to malfunction.

"Every time she sneezes, I wake up and nudge her to see if she's all right," Ofenbeck says. "Sneezes are scary".

A year after the rupture, Van Patten flew to Nashville for specialized surgery to ensure she would have a strong voice for her return to television part-time in June 1998. She wore wigs on camera as her shaved hair grew up and plans to do the same this time around.

The only thing about (being bald) was I got cold," she says. Ofenbeck took her on a shopping trip to Target where she bought ten hats-mostly baseball caps, but a few dressy velvet hats and bandanas mixed in. Problem solved.

Her most recent foray into the operating room was more than a simple shunt revision. Alvarez put an endoscope -a tube with a camera and light attached to one end-into the third ventricle of her brain. There he found a golf ball sized cyst, opened it and removed the fluid within. He says the aneurysm's rupture caused blood to spill out into the brain and scar its covering. That led to trapped fluid and the formation of the cyst. "Since they took that out, I can tell a difference," Van Patten says. "My tongue was partially paralyzed. It's not anymore."

Van Patten and her husband have maintained strong spirits. While the doctors prohibited scuba diving-she's been certified a week before this happened-roller coaster riding-something the couple loved to do-or weight lifting, Ofenbeck says he doesn't try to limit her other actions.

"She can function," he says. "I certainly don't try to put any restrictions on what she does."

Ofenbeck says the aneurysm has changed his wife in unexpected ways. She'd gone to college on a golf scholarship but now has no desire to pick up her clubs. Her handwriting is also different. And while her long-term memory remains clear, her short term memory has disappeared. The endoscopic surgery has given them hope it might improve because the cyst was pressing on that part of her brain. Alvarez expects continued improvement in the memory areas affected by the cyst-but that doesn't include all memory damaged by the initial rupture.

In the meantime, they simply deal with whatever Van Patten's brain throws at them. Ofenbeck has noticed that anywhere from five to 30 minutes after they discuss something, she forgets it. Four to five weeks later, it reappears in her mind.

Dealing with memory loss is frustrating for both of them.

"She'll ask how was work? Six times a night," he says. "You have to not get frustrated when you get the repetitive question. it's a mental battle for me as well as her."

Van Patten didn't know she had a memory problem until Ofenbeck pointed out her repetition.

'Now that I'm aware of that, its hard," she says. "I think before I say anything, 'did I already say that?'"

When Van Patten realizes she has repeated herself and gets flustered, her husband cuts her off mid-apology with a gentle squeeze to her shoulder, affectionately reminding her there's never a need to say she's sorry.

Ofenbeck bought her an electronic organizer so she can keep track of her schedule. And Van Patten has learned little tricks that help, such as writing down where she parks when she goes to the mall.

"I look at the big picture," Ofenbeck says. "I'll Answer her question 70 times as long as she's here to ask it."

Van Patten expects to feel well enough to return to work within the next month and is determined to meet the challenge.

"I tend to get overwhelmed easily by things that have a lot of details." she says. "I need to step back, concentrate, and focus. It's extremely frustrating and I have no patience. It's very discouraging at times."

Dangling from a chain around Ofenbeck's neck is a tiny metal aneurysm clip identical to the one used to close the hemorrhage during her first surgery.

"That's what I have in my head," she says holding it up. "It is like a good luck charm."

Success Gets Redefined-by Dayna Harpster Fort Myers News Press-Dec 13,2011

A former TV anchor and her husband reframe their lives and measure her progress by her medical strides

Todd Ofenbeck sits on a couch facing the camera, legs turned slightly to the left and toward his wife, Amy beside him. In the video shot shortly after she suffered a burst aneurysm at the base of her brain, the young woman looks thin, pale, and as fragile as a baby bird. She wears a baseball cap over recently sprouted hair, lingering evidence of the first of what would be eight brain surgeries over the next 14 years. Her voice is a whisper due to a paralyzed vocal cord.

The clip that follows-featuring her as a TV anchorwoman, which described her for most of the day on July 15, 1997-was recorded mere months but actually a lifetime earlier. The bleeding in her brain that July day changed absolutely everything. As reporter Amy Van Patten she dominates the screen, making Amy Ofenbeck appear small. But most resonant in retrospect is Todd's statement about the couple being newlyweds. They say the first year is the hardest, he says. "But if we can make it through this first year, we can make it through anything."

And they have.

He couldn't even spell aneurysm back then, Todd says. And doctors had to explain to both of them what happened. Some details are crystalline; Todd remembers being pulled aside near the emergency room by a hospital liaison "as clear as day". Amy remembers reading his notes from that day."You wrote 50/50," she reminded him one evening at their Edison Park home, seated at the dining table on which was a salt and pepper set in the shape of a brain. There are light moments.

Today Amy is 41, Todd 42, and as the director of photojournalism for Waterman Broadcasting, he is the one who goes to the station every day. She works part time in the public relations department for Goodwill, where she was named Achiever of the Year in 2005.

They point to different milestones in their lives together than they once imagined. Before that day, the two very career oriented television journalists were embracing a move from their roots in the Midwest to jobs in Southwest Florida and higher profiles. Todd was behind the camera and Amy in front and both assumed she would be leading the way toward life's bigger markets.

But that was before she slumped over a weight machine at a Southwest Florida gym, besieged by what her neurologist said was one of the worst brain hemorrhages he had seen in 26 years of practice. "Remarkable that she survived," he said on the same video clip, reported by WZVN TV Fort Myers colleague Emily Norman in 1997 and shared with Amy's first audience as a professional, WSIL in Carterville, IL.

Milestones today are measured not in ratings numbers but in strides made as a rider at Special Equestrians, where Amy improves her balance with help from its horses and therapeutic team. Success is gauged by how many patients she and her dog, Gillespie, see as a therapy team at Lee Memorial Hospital, and by how many young readers are nurtured along in a Lee County schools program that brings special dogs-and their special people-into the classroom.

Progress today is also measured by her ability to move through a continuous string of unexpected challenged, such as severe malfunctions with the shunt that drains excess fluid from her brain, a cyst forming on her spine and further complicating her brain injury and one period she still does not like to think about, when she said repeated brain traumas triggered delusions and psychosis.

She still has short term memory deficit, she said. She sometimes asks Todd the same question multiple times. That's when the answer to "Gee, how many times do I have to tell you..." is "Well one more."

They did not have children. It would have been high risk, Amy said. They hadn't gotten to that point in their lives before her injury and think they may have remained a two-person family anyway.

One thing hasn't changed a bit, Todd said. She's still a news junkie. And Amy smiled.

TV Reporter Battles Illness-Dave Taylor Naples Daily News

At age 27, Amy Van Patten had a bright future in the television business. She was attractive, an accomplished anchor and working in the same business with her husband after moving to Southwest Florida from the Paducah, KY market. She was enjoying the sun, warm weather and in laws who lived nearby.

Now, the WZVN-TV reporter is contemplating her next move after suffering numerous brain operations that have her wondering about her career.

Amy had been on the job at the local ABC affiliate for just more than six months in July 1997, when she was working out and collapsed at a local fitness center. She was rushed to the hospital and told she had suffered an aneurysm. She underwent her first brain operation and the aneurysm was clipped.

Amy was confined to the hospital for two months before beginning rehabilitation. One of her vocal cords had been paralyzed. She wasn't doing well. Doctors determined a ventricle in her brain had shifted. Another operation inserted a shunt in the ventricle and there would be three more procedures for revisions.

A feeding tube had to be inserted in her stomach for nourishment. Because of the paralysis to her vocal cord, she could only whisper. An operation at Vanderbilt University required her to train her repaired vocal cord to be able to eat.

After feeling better Amy tried to return to the world of local television news.

"I tried to go back to work too soon," she says. Amy found out another brain operation would be required.

Amy now knows enough about medical procedures to write a book. She is currently on disability trying to decide her next step. Yet she remains optimistic.

"I've had my bad days and it hasn't been easy, ' she says with noticeable energy in her voice. "The last surgery really wiped me out." Amy says she is going to fully recover before deciding if she will return to television news or try another occupation. She says station management and co-workers have been very supportive.

The aneurysm was a birth defect most people don't suffer until they are 40 or 50 years of age.

“Reporting is a very stressful business, which I never realized before,” she says. “I really don’t know how I’ve been able to keep everything in perspective. I think its taken several years for everything to really sink in. What choice do I have? I was dealt these cards I might as well play them. Its been an incredible learning experience for me and my family”.

Brain Aneurysm Challenging, Even Years Later
JL Watson
Lee Memorial Health System newsletter

She was young and a newly-wed with a brand new job in a new city and state. Television reporter Amy Ofenbeck was making a fresh start when she moved to Folrt Myers in 1996. Just seven months later, her life changed dramatically.

"I was working out at the gym and I collapsed," Amy says. "I had a brain aneurysm. Until that point I was perfectly healthy and had no idea. I did not have headaches or any other signs that something was wrong."

Amy spent nine weeks in the hospital and completed rehabilitation. Even so, she developed headaches and some memory problems. Fluid buildup on her brain led to another surgery to install a shunt to drain the excess fluid. She would need 4 shunt revisions because of complications. The seventh and final surgery was for a cyst in her spine the result of something called Chiari Malformation.

"It was a tough time," Amy says. Even so, she kept moving forward with her life. She gave up her broadcasting career, but found new opportunities working for Goodwill Industries. Despite several challenges, including balance problems that have required the use of a cane, Amy resumed driving, playing with her dogs and is writing a book about her experience.

For several years Amy thought her medical issues were mostly in the past, until last year. "I fell in the bathroom and tried for nine hours to crawl to the phone," she says. "My husband was out of town. He kept calling and so did my parents."

She dialed 911 and paramedics arrived within minutes. Despite sustaining some bruises, she was uninjured. CAT scans revealed no cause for the fall. She spent three days in the hospital and a month in physical therapy.

"I'm still limited in what I can do," Amy says. "But it makes me slow down and appreciate the little things."

A brain injury like Amy had often cannot be explained, says she neurosurgeon Gary J Correnti MD. "A brain aneurysm usually occurs at a branch-point of an artery," Dr Correnti says. "There tends to be a weak spot in the blood vessel in that area. High blood pressure and smoking are two risk factors associated with aneurysm formation. In Amy's case, it was a naturally occurring weak spot.

Most people with an aneurysm are not aware of their condition until the aneurysm ruptures. "At that time it has been described as causing 'the worst headache in my life' " Dr Correnti says. After surviving the initial rupture, Amy was able to have surgery to prevent a second hemorrhage and near-certain death.

"Amy's strength and determination enabled her to overcome several post-hemorrhage complications, including hydrocephalus," Dr Correnti says. "She worked very hard in physical and occupational therapy, and it shows in her continued progress. I am very proud of her independence and progress."

www.ingramcontent.com/pod-product-compliance
Lightning Source LLC
Chambersburg PA
CBHW030520290526
45786CB00004B/1547
9781522963141